This book belongs to:

Week Starting _3/8/21_

Monday

Time	Pace	Distance	HR
8:35 Am.	17 min P. mile	@ 3 mile	

Weather	Calories	Shoes	Other
Cold clear		Hiking Shoes	

Route		Run Type	
Fair haven bike Path			

Tuesday

Time	Pace	Distance	HR
8:36	17 min P. mile	@ 3 miles	

Weather	Calories	Shoes	Other
Clear. warmer		Hiking	

Route		Run Type	

Wednesday

Time	Pace	Distance	HR
10 - 11:15		3.34 miles	

Weather	Calories	Shoes	Other
clear			

Route		Run Type	

Thursday

Time	Pace	Distance	HR

Weather	Calories	Shoes	Other

Route		Run Type	

Friday

Time	Pace	Distance	HR
Weather	Calories	Shoes	Other
Route		Run Type	

Saturday

Time	Pace	Distance	HR
Weather	Calories	Shoes	Other
Route		Run Type	

Sunday

Time	Pace	Distance	HR
Weather	Calories	Shoes	Other
Route		Run Type	

Notes

Week Starting _____

Monday			
Time	Pace	Distance	HR
Weather	Calories	Shoes	Other
Route		Run Type	

Tuesday			
Time	Pace	Distance	HR
Weather	Calories	Shoes	Other
Route		Run Type	

Wednesday			
Time	Pace	Distance	HR
Weather	Calories	Shoes	Other
Route		Run Type	

Thursday			
Time	Pace	Distance	HR
Weather	Calories	Shoes	Other
Route		Run Type	

Friday			
Time	Pace	Distance	HR
Weather	Calories	Shoes	Other
Route		Run Type	

Saturday			
Time	Pace	Distance	HR
Weather	Calories	Shoes	Other
Route		Run Type	

Sunday			
Time	Pace	Distance	HR
Weather	Calories	Shoes	Other
Route		Run Type	

Notes

Week Starting _____

Monday

Time	Pace	Distance	HR
Weather	Calories	Shoes	Other
Route		Run Type	

Tuesday

Time	Pace	Distance	HR
Weather	Calories	Shoes	Other
Route		Run Type	

Wednesday

Time	Pace	Distance	HR
Weather	Calories	Shoes	Other
Route		Run Type	

Thursday

Time	Pace	Distance	HR
Weather	Calories	Shoes	Other
Route		Run Type	

Friday

Time	Pace	Distance	HR
Weather	Calories	Shoes	Other
Route		Run Type	

Saturday

Time	Pace	Distance	HR
Weather	Calories	Shoes	Other
Route		Run Type	

Sunday

Time	Pace	Distance	HR
Weather	Calories	Shoes	Other
Route		Run Type	

Notes

Week Starting _____

Monday			
Time	Pace	Distance	HR
Weather	Calories	Shoes	Other
Route		Run Type	

Tuesday			
Time	Pace	Distance	HR
Weather	Calories	Shoes	Other
Route		Run Type	

Wednesday			
Time	Pace	Distance	HR
Weather	Calories	Shoes	Other
Route		Run Type	

Thursday			
Time	Pace	Distance	HR
Weather	Calories	Shoes	Other
Route		Run Type	

Friday			
Time	Pace	Distance	HR
Weather	Calories	Shoes	Other
Route		Run Type	

Saturday			
Time	Pace	Distance	HR
Weather	Calories	Shoes	Other
Route		Run Type	

Sunday			
Time	Pace	Distance	HR
Weather	Calories	Shoes	Other
Route		Run Type	

Notes

Week Starting _____

Monday

Time	Pace	Distance	HR
Weather	Calories	Shoes	Other
Route		Run Type	

Tuesday

Time	Pace	Distance	HR
Weather	Calories	Shoes	Other
Route		Run Type	

Wednesday

Time	Pace	Distance	HR
Weather	Calories	Shoes	Other
Route		Run Type	

Thursday

Time	Pace	Distance	HR
Weather	Calories	Shoes	Other
Route		Run Type	

Friday

Time	Pace	Distance	HR
Weather	Calories	Shoes	Other
Route		Run Type	

Saturday

Time	Pace	Distance	HR
Weather	Calories	Shoes	Other
Route		Run Type	

Sunday

Time	Pace	Distance	HR
Weather	Calories	Shoes	Other
Route		Run Type	

Notes

Week Starting _____

Monday			
Time	Pace	Distance	HR
Weather	Calories	Shoes	Other
Route		Run Type	

Tuesday			
Time	Pace	Distance	HR
Weather	Calories	Shoes	Other
Route		Run Type	

Wednesday			
Time	Pace	Distance	HR
Weather	Calories	Shoes	Other
Route		Run Type	

Thursday			
Time	Pace	Distance	HR
Weather	Calories	Shoes	Other
Route		Run Type	

Friday			
Time	Pace	Distance	HR
Weather	Calories	Shoes	Other
Route		Run Type	

Saturday			
Time	Pace	Distance	HR
Weather	Calories	Shoes	Other
Route		Run Type	

Sunday			
Time	Pace	Distance	HR
Weather	Calories	Shoes	Other
Route		Run Type	

Notes

Week Starting _____

Monday

Time	Pace	Distance	HR
Weather	Calories	Shoes	Other
Route		Run Type	

Tuesday

Time	Pace	Distance	HR
Weather	Calories	Shoes	Other
Route		Run Type	

Wednesday

Time	Pace	Distance	HR
Weather	Calories	Shoes	Other
Route		Run Type	

Thursday

Time	Pace	Distance	HR
Weather	Calories	Shoes	Other
Route		Run Type	

Friday

Time	Pace	Distance	HR
Weather	Calories	Shoes	Other
Route		Run Type	

Saturday

Time	Pace	Distance	HR
Weather	Calories	Shoes	Other
Route		Run Type	

Sunday

Time	Pace	Distance	HR
Weather	Calories	Shoes	Other
Route		Run Type	

Notes

Week Starting _____

Monday			
Time	Pace	Distance	HR
Weather	Calories	Shoes	Other
Route		Run Type	

Tuesday			
Time	Pace	Distance	HR
Weather	Calories	Shoes	Other
Route		Run Type	

Wednesday			
Time	Pace	Distance	HR
Weather	Calories	Shoes	Other
Route		Run Type	

Thursday			
Time	Pace	Distance	HR
Weather	Calories	Shoes	Other
Route		Run Type	

Friday			
Time	Pace	Distance	HR
Weather	Calories	Shoes	Other
Route		Run Type	

Saturday			
Time	Pace	Distance	HR
Weather	Calories	Shoes	Other
Route		Run Type	

Sunday			
Time	Pace	Distance	HR
Weather	Calories	Shoes	Other
Route		Run Type	

Notes

Week Starting _____

Monday

Time	Pace	Distance	HR
Weather	Calories	Shoes	Other
Route		Run Type	

Tuesday

Time	Pace	Distance	HR
Weather	Calories	Shoes	Other
Route		Run Type	

Wednesday

Time	Pace	Distance	HR
Weather	Calories	Shoes	Other
Route		Run Type	

Thursday

Time	Pace	Distance	HR
Weather	Calories	Shoes	Other
Route		Run Type	

Friday			
Time	Pace	Distance	HR
Weather	Calories	Shoes	Other
Route		Run Type	

Saturday			
Time	Pace	Distance	HR
Weather	Calories	Shoes	Other
Route		Run Type	

Sunday			
Time	Pace	Distance	HR
Weather	Calories	Shoes	Other
Route		Run Type	

Notes

Week Starting _____

Monday			
Time	Pace	Distance	HR
Weather	Calories	Shoes	Other
Route		Run Type	

Tuesday			
Time	Pace	Distance	HR
Weather	Calories	Shoes	Other
Route		Run Type	

Wednesday			
Time	Pace	Distance	HR
Weather	Calories	Shoes	Other
Route		Run Type	

Thursday			
Time	Pace	Distance	HR
Weather	Calories	Shoes	Other
Route		Run Type	

Friday			
Time	Pace	Distance	HR
Weather	Calories	Shoes	Other
Route		Run Type	

Saturday			
Time	Pace	Distance	HR
Weather	Calories	Shoes	Other
Route		Run Type	

Sunday			
Time	Pace	Distance	HR
Weather	Calories	Shoes	Other
Route		Run Type	

Notes

Week Starting _____

Monday			
Time	Pace	Distance	HR
Weather	Calories	Shoes	Other
Route		Run Type	

Tuesday			
Time	Pace	Distance	HR
Weather	Calories	Shoes	Other
Route		Run Type	

Wednesday			
Time	Pace	Distance	HR
Weather	Calories	Shoes	Other
Route		Run Type	

Thursday			
Time	Pace	Distance	HR
Weather	Calories	Shoes	Other
Route		Run Type	

Friday			
Time	Pace	Distance	HR
Weather	Calories	Shoes	Other
Route		Run Type	

Saturday			
Time	Pace	Distance	HR
Weather	Calories	Shoes	Other
Route		Run Type	

Sunday			
Time	Pace	Distance	HR
Weather	Calories	Shoes	Other
Route		Run Type	

Notes

Week Starting _____

Monday			
Time	Pace	Distance	HR
Weather	Calories	Shoes	Other
Route		Run Type	

Tuesday			
Time	Pace	Distance	HR
Weather	Calories	Shoes	Other
Route		Run Type	

Wednesday			
Time	Pace	Distance	HR
Weather	Calories	Shoes	Other
Route		Run Type	

Thursday			
Time	Pace	Distance	HR
Weather	Calories	Shoes	Other
Route		Run Type	

Friday

Time	Pace	Distance	HR
Weather	Calories	Shoes	Other
Route		Run Type	

Saturday

Time	Pace	Distance	HR
Weather	Calories	Shoes	Other
Route		Run Type	

Sunday

Time	Pace	Distance	HR
Weather	Calories	Shoes	Other
Route		Run Type	

Notes

Week Starting _____

Monday			
Time	Pace	Distance	HR
Weather	Calories	Shoes	Other
Route		Run Type	

Tuesday			
Time	Pace	Distance	HR
Weather	Calories	Shoes	Other
Route		Run Type	

Wednesday			
Time	Pace	Distance	HR
Weather	Calories	Shoes	Other
Route		Run Type	

Thursday			
Time	Pace	Distance	HR
Weather	Calories	Shoes	Other
Route		Run Type	

Friday			
Time	Pace	Distance	HR
Weather	Calories	Shoes	Other
Route		Run Type	

Saturday			
Time	Pace	Distance	HR
Weather	Calories	Shoes	Other
Route		Run Type	

Sunday			
Time	Pace	Distance	HR
Weather	Calories	Shoes	Other
Route		Run Type	

Notes

Week Starting _____

Monday			
Time	Pace	Distance	HR
Weather	Calories	Shoes	Other
Route		Run Type	

Tuesday			
Time	Pace	Distance	HR
Weather	Calories	Shoes	Other
Route		Run Type	

Wednesday			
Time	Pace	Distance	HR
Weather	Calories	Shoes	Other
Route		Run Type	

Thursday			
Time	Pace	Distance	HR
Weather	Calories	Shoes	Other
Route		Run Type	

Friday

Time	Pace	Distance	HR
Weather	Calories	Shoes	Other
Route		Run Type	

Saturday

Time	Pace	Distance	HR
Weather	Calories	Shoes	Other
Route		Run Type	

Sunday

Time	Pace	Distance	HR
Weather	Calories	Shoes	Other
Route		Run Type	

Notes

Week Starting _____

Monday

Time	Pace	Distance	HR
Weather	Calories	Shoes	Other
Route		Run Type	

Tuesday

Time	Pace	Distance	HR
Weather	Calories	Shoes	Other
Route		Run Type	

Wednesday

Time	Pace	Distance	HR
Weather	Calories	Shoes	Other
Route		Run Type	

Thursday

Time	Pace	Distance	HR
Weather	Calories	Shoes	Other
Route		Run Type	

Friday

Time	Pace	Distance	HR
Weather	Calories	Shoes	Other
Route		Run Type	

Saturday

Time	Pace	Distance	HR
Weather	Calories	Shoes	Other
Route		Run Type	

Sunday

Time	Pace	Distance	HR
Weather	Calories	Shoes	Other
Route		Run Type	

Notes

Week Starting _____

Monday			
Time	Pace	Distance	HR
Weather	Calories	Shoes	Other
Route		Run Type	

Tuesday			
Time	Pace	Distance	HR
Weather	Calories	Shoes	Other
Route		Run Type	

Wednesday			
Time	Pace	Distance	HR
Weather	Calories	Shoes	Other
Route		Run Type	

Thursday			
Time	Pace	Distance	HR
Weather	Calories	Shoes	Other
Route		Run Type	

Friday

Time	Pace	Distance	HR
Weather	Calories	Shoes	Other
Route		Run Type	

Saturday

Time	Pace	Distance	HR
Weather	Calories	Shoes	Other
Route		Run Type	

Sunday

Time	Pace	Distance	HR
Weather	Calories	Shoes	Other
Route		Run Type	

Notes

Week Starting _____

Monday			
Time	Pace	Distance	HR
Weather	Calories	Shoes	Other
Route		Run Type	

Tuesday			
Time	Pace	Distance	HR
Weather	Calories	Shoes	Other
Route		Run Type	

Wednesday			
Time	Pace	Distance	HR
Weather	Calories	Shoes	Other
Route		Run Type	

Thursday			
Time	Pace	Distance	HR
Weather	Calories	Shoes	Other
Route		Run Type	

Friday

Time	Pace	Distance	HR
Weather	Calories	Shoes	Other
Route		Run Type	

Saturday

Time	Pace	Distance	HR
Weather	Calories	Shoes	Other
Route		Run Type	

Sunday

Time	Pace	Distance	HR
Weather	Calories	Shoes	Other
Route		Run Type	

Notes

Week Starting _____

Monday			
Time	Pace	Distance	HR
Weather	Calories	Shoes	Other
Route		Run Type	

Tuesday			
Time	Pace	Distance	HR
Weather	Calories	Shoes	Other
Route		Run Type	

Wednesday			
Time	Pace	Distance	HR
Weather	Calories	Shoes	Other
Route		Run Type	

Thursday			
Time	Pace	Distance	HR
Weather	Calories	Shoes	Other
Route		Run Type	

Friday

Time	Pace	Distance	HR
Weather	Calories	Shoes	Other
Route		Run Type	

Saturday

Time	Pace	Distance	HR
Weather	Calories	Shoes	Other
Route		Run Type	

Sunday

Time	Pace	Distance	HR
Weather	Calories	Shoes	Other
Route		Run Type	

Notes

Week Starting _____

Monday			
Time	Pace	Distance	HR
Weather	Calories	Shoes	Other
Route		Run Type	

Tuesday			
Time	Pace	Distance	HR
Weather	Calories	Shoes	Other
Route		Run Type	

Wednesday			
Time	Pace	Distance	HR
Weather	Calories	Shoes	Other
Route		Run Type	

Thursday			
Time	Pace	Distance	HR
Weather	Calories	Shoes	Other
Route		Run Type	

Friday			
Time	Pace	Distance	HR
Weather	Calories	Shoes	Other
Route		Run Type	

Saturday			
Time	Pace	Distance	HR
Weather	Calories	Shoes	Other
Route		Run Type	

Sunday			
Time	Pace	Distance	HR
Weather	Calories	Shoes	Other
Route		Run Type	

Notes

Week Starting _____

Monday			
Time	Pace	Distance	HR
Weather	Calories	Shoes	Other
Route		Run Type	

Tuesday			
Time	Pace	Distance	HR
Weather	Calories	Shoes	Other
Route		Run Type	

Wednesday			
Time	Pace	Distance	HR
Weather	Calories	Shoes	Other
Route		Run Type	

Thursday			
Time	Pace	Distance	HR
Weather	Calories	Shoes	Other
Route		Run Type	

Friday

Time	Pace	Distance	HR
Weather	Calories	Shoes	Other
Route		Run Type	

Saturday

Time	Pace	Distance	HR
Weather	Calories	Shoes	Other
Route		Run Type	

Sunday

Time	Pace	Distance	HR
Weather	Calories	Shoes	Other
Route		Run Type	

Notes

Week Starting _____

Monday			
Time	Pace	Distance	HR
Weather	Calories	Shoes	Other
Route		Run Type	

Tuesday			
Time	Pace	Distance	HR
Weather	Calories	Shoes	Other
Route		Run Type	

Wednesday			
Time	Pace	Distance	HR
Weather	Calories	Shoes	Other
Route		Run Type	

Thursday			
Time	Pace	Distance	HR
Weather	Calories	Shoes	Other
Route		Run Type	

Friday

Time	Pace	Distance	HR
Weather	Calories	Shoes	Other
Route		Run Type	

Saturday

Time	Pace	Distance	HR
Weather	Calories	Shoes	Other
Route		Run Type	

Sunday

Time	Pace	Distance	HR
Weather	Calories	Shoes	Other
Route		Run Type	

Notes

Week Starting _____

Monday

Time	Pace	Distance	HR
Weather	Calories	Shoes	Other
Route		Run Type	

Tuesday

Time	Pace	Distance	HR
Weather	Calories	Shoes	Other
Route		Run Type	

Wednesday

Time	Pace	Distance	HR
Weather	Calories	Shoes	Other
Route		Run Type	

Thursday

Time	Pace	Distance	HR
Weather	Calories	Shoes	Other
Route		Run Type	

Friday			
Time	Pace	Distance	HR
Weather	Calories	Shoes	Other
Route		Run Type	

Saturday			
Time	Pace	Distance	HR
Weather	Calories	Shoes	Other
Route		Run Type	

Sunday			
Time	Pace	Distance	HR
Weather	Calories	Shoes	Other
Route		Run Type	

Notes

Week Starting _____

Monday			
Time	Pace	Distance	HR
Weather	Calories	Shoes	Other
Route		Run Type	

Tuesday			
Time	Pace	Distance	HR
Weather	Calories	Shoes	Other
Route		Run Type	

Wednesday			
Time	Pace	Distance	HR
Weather	Calories	Shoes	Other
Route		Run Type	

Thursday			
Time	Pace	Distance	HR
Weather	Calories	Shoes	Other
Route		Run Type	

Friday

Time	Pace	Distance	HR
Weather	Calories	Shoes	Other
Route		Run Type	

Saturday

Time	Pace	Distance	HR
Weather	Calories	Shoes	Other
Route		Run Type	

Sunday

Time	Pace	Distance	HR
Weather	Calories	Shoes	Other
Route		Run Type	

Notes

Week Starting _____

Monday			
Time	Pace	Distance	HR
Weather	Calories	Shoes	Other
Route		Run Type	

Tuesday			
Time	Pace	Distance	HR
Weather	Calories	Shoes	Other
Route		Run Type	

Wednesday			
Time	Pace	Distance	HR
Weather	Calories	Shoes	Other
Route		Run Type	

Thursday			
Time	Pace	Distance	HR
Weather	Calories	Shoes	Other
Route		Run Type	

Friday			
Time	Pace	Distance	HR
Weather	Calories	Shoes	Other
Route		Run Type	

Saturday			
Time	Pace	Distance	HR
Weather	Calories	Shoes	Other
Route		Run Type	

Sunday			
Time	Pace	Distance	HR
Weather	Calories	Shoes	Other
Route		Run Type	

Notes

Week Starting _____

Monday

Time	Pace	Distance	HR
Weather	Calories	Shoes	Other
Route		Run Type	

Tuesday

Time	Pace	Distance	HR
Weather	Calories	Shoes	Other
Route		Run Type	

Wednesday

Time	Pace	Distance	HR
Weather	Calories	Shoes	Other
Route		Run Type	

Thursday

Time	Pace	Distance	HR
Weather	Calories	Shoes	Other
Route		Run Type	

Friday			
Time	Pace	Distance	HR
Weather	Calories	Shoes	Other
Route		Run Type	

Saturday			
Time	Pace	Distance	HR
Weather	Calories	Shoes	Other
Route		Run Type	

Sunday			
Time	Pace	Distance	HR
Weather	Calories	Shoes	Other
Route		Run Type	

Notes

Week Starting _____

Monday			
Time	Pace	Distance	HR
Weather	Calories	Shoes	Other
Route		Run Type	

Tuesday			
Time	Pace	Distance	HR
Weather	Calories	Shoes	Other
Route		Run Type	

Wednesday			
Time	Pace	Distance	HR
Weather	Calories	Shoes	Other
Route		Run Type	

Thursday			
Time	Pace	Distance	HR
Weather	Calories	Shoes	Other
Route		Run Type	

Friday			
Time	Pace	Distance	HR
Weather	Calories	Shoes	Other
Route		Run Type	

Saturday			
Time	Pace	Distance	HR
Weather	Calories	Shoes	Other
Route		Run Type	

Sunday			
Time	Pace	Distance	HR
Weather	Calories	Shoes	Other
Route		Run Type	

Notes

Week Starting _____

Monday			
Time	Pace	Distance	HR
Weather	Calories	Shoes	Other
Route		Run Type	

Tuesday			
Time	Pace	Distance	HR
Weather	Calories	Shoes	Other
Route		Run Type	

Wednesday			
Time	Pace	Distance	HR
Weather	Calories	Shoes	Other
Route		Run Type	

Thursday			
Time	Pace	Distance	HR
Weather	Calories	Shoes	Other
Route		Run Type	

Friday

Time	Pace	Distance	HR
Weather	Calories	Shoes	Other
Route		Run Type	

Saturday

Time	Pace	Distance	HR
Weather	Calories	Shoes	Other
Route		Run Type	

Sunday

Time	Pace	Distance	HR
Weather	Calories	Shoes	Other
Route		Run Type	

Notes

Week Starting _____

Monday			
Time	Pace	Distance	HR
Weather	Calories	Shoes	Other
Route		Run Type	

Tuesday			
Time	Pace	Distance	HR
Weather	Calories	Shoes	Other
Route		Run Type	

Wednesday			
Time	Pace	Distance	HR
Weather	Calories	Shoes	Other
Route		Run Type	

Thursday			
Time	Pace	Distance	HR
Weather	Calories	Shoes	Other
Route		Run Type	

Friday			
Time	Pace	Distance	HR
Weather	Calories	Shoes	Other
Route		Run Type	

Saturday			
Time	Pace	Distance	HR
Weather	Calories	Shoes	Other
Route		Run Type	

Sunday			
Time	Pace	Distance	HR
Weather	Calories	Shoes	Other
Route		Run Type	

Notes

Week Starting _____

Monday			
Time	Pace	Distance	HR
Weather	Calories	Shoes	Other
Route		Run Type	

Tuesday			
Time	Pace	Distance	HR
Weather	Calories	Shoes	Other
Route		Run Type	

Wednesday			
Time	Pace	Distance	HR
Weather	Calories	Shoes	Other
Route		Run Type	

Thursday			
Time	Pace	Distance	HR
Weather	Calories	Shoes	Other
Route		Run Type	

Friday			
Time	Pace	Distance	HR
Weather	Calories	Shoes	Other
Route		Run Type	

Saturday			
Time	Pace	Distance	HR
Weather	Calories	Shoes	Other
Route		Run Type	

Sunday			
Time	Pace	Distance	HR
Weather	Calories	Shoes	Other
Route		Run Type	

Notes

Week Starting _____

Monday			
Time	Pace	Distance	HR
Weather	Calories	Shoes	Other
Route		Run Type	

Tuesday			
Time	Pace	Distance	HR
Weather	Calories	Shoes	Other
Route		Run Type	

Wednesday			
Time	Pace	Distance	HR
Weather	Calories	Shoes	Other
Route		Run Type	

Thursday			
Time	Pace	Distance	HR
Weather	Calories	Shoes	Other
Route		Run Type	

Friday

Time	Pace	Distance	HR
Weather	Calories	Shoes	Other
Route		Run Type	

Saturday

Time	Pace	Distance	HR
Weather	Calories	Shoes	Other
Route		Run Type	

Sunday

Time	Pace	Distance	HR
Weather	Calories	Shoes	Other
Route		Run Type	

Notes

Week Starting _____

Monday			
Time	Pace	Distance	HR
Weather	Calories	Shoes	Other
Route		Run Type	

Tuesday			
Time	Pace	Distance	HR
Weather	Calories	Shoes	Other
Route		Run Type	

Wednesday			
Time	Pace	Distance	HR
Weather	Calories	Shoes	Other
Route		Run Type	

Thursday			
Time	Pace	Distance	HR
Weather	Calories	Shoes	Other
Route		Run Type	

Friday			
Time	Pace	Distance	HR
Weather	Calories	Shoes	Other
Route		Run Type	

Saturday			
Time	Pace	Distance	HR
Weather	Calories	Shoes	Other
Route		Run Type	

Sunday			
Time	Pace	Distance	HR
Weather	Calories	Shoes	Other
Route		Run Type	

Notes

Week Starting _____

Monday			
Time	Pace	Distance	HR
Weather	Calories	Shoes	Other
Route		Run Type	

Tuesday			
Time	Pace	Distance	HR
Weather	Calories	Shoes	Other
Route		Run Type	

Wednesday			
Time	Pace	Distance	HR
Weather	Calories	Shoes	Other
Route		Run Type	

Thursday			
Time	Pace	Distance	HR
Weather	Calories	Shoes	Other
Route		Run Type	

Friday			
Time	Pace	Distance	HR
Weather	Calories	Shoes	Other
Route		Run Type	

Saturday			
Time	Pace	Distance	HR
Weather	Calories	Shoes	Other
Route		Run Type	

Sunday			
Time	Pace	Distance	HR
Weather	Calories	Shoes	Other
Route		Run Type	

Notes

Week Starting _____

Monday			
Time	Pace	Distance	HR
Weather	Calories	Shoes	Other
Route		Run Type	

Tuesday			
Time	Pace	Distance	HR
Weather	Calories	Shoes	Other
Route		Run Type	

Wednesday			
Time	Pace	Distance	HR
Weather	Calories	Shoes	Other
Route		Run Type	

Thursday			
Time	Pace	Distance	HR
Weather	Calories	Shoes	Other
Route		Run Type	

Friday

Time	Pace	Distance	HR
Weather	Calories	Shoes	Other
Route		Run Type	

Saturday

Time	Pace	Distance	HR
Weather	Calories	Shoes	Other
Route		Run Type	

Sunday

Time	Pace	Distance	HR
Weather	Calories	Shoes	Other
Route		Run Type	

Notes

Week Starting _____

Monday			
Time	Pace	Distance	HR
Weather	Calories	Shoes	Other
Route		Run Type	

Tuesday			
Time	Pace	Distance	HR
Weather	Calories	Shoes	Other
Route		Run Type	

Wednesday			
Time	Pace	Distance	HR
Weather	Calories	Shoes	Other
Route		Run Type	

Thursday			
Time	Pace	Distance	HR
Weather	Calories	Shoes	Other
Route		Run Type	

Friday

Time	Pace	Distance	HR
Weather	Calories	Shoes	Other
Route		Run Type	

Saturday

Time	Pace	Distance	HR
Weather	Calories	Shoes	Other
Route		Run Type	

Sunday

Time	Pace	Distance	HR
Weather	Calories	Shoes	Other
Route		Run Type	

Notes

Week Starting _____

Monday			
Time	Pace	Distance	HR
Weather	Calories	Shoes	Other
Route		Run Type	

Tuesday			
Time	Pace	Distance	HR
Weather	Calories	Shoes	Other
Route		Run Type	

Wednesday			
Time	Pace	Distance	HR
Weather	Calories	Shoes	Other
Route		Run Type	

Thursday			
Time	Pace	Distance	HR
Weather	Calories	Shoes	Other
Route		Run Type	

Friday			
Time	Pace	Distance	HR
Weather	Calories	Shoes	Other
Route		Run Type	

Saturday			
Time	Pace	Distance	HR
Weather	Calories	Shoes	Other
Route		Run Type	

Sunday			
Time	Pace	Distance	HR
Weather	Calories	Shoes	Other
Route		Run Type	

Notes

Week Starting _____

Monday			
Time	Pace	Distance	HR
Weather	Calories	Shoes	Other
Route		Run Type	

Tuesday			
Time	Pace	Distance	HR
Weather	Calories	Shoes	Other
Route		Run Type	

Wednesday			
Time	Pace	Distance	HR
Weather	Calories	Shoes	Other
Route		Run Type	

Thursday			
Time	Pace	Distance	HR
Weather	Calories	Shoes	Other
Route		Run Type	

Friday

Time	Pace	Distance	HR
Weather	Calories	Shoes	Other
Route		Run Type	

Saturday

Time	Pace	Distance	HR
Weather	Calories	Shoes	Other
Route		Run Type	

Sunday

Time	Pace	Distance	HR
Weather	Calories	Shoes	Other
Route		Run Type	

Notes

Week Starting _____

Monday			
Time	Pace	Distance	HR
Weather	Calories	Shoes	Other
Route		Run Type	

Tuesday			
Time	Pace	Distance	HR
Weather	Calories	Shoes	Other
Route		Run Type	

Wednesday			
Time	Pace	Distance	HR
Weather	Calories	Shoes	Other
Route		Run Type	

Thursday			
Time	Pace	Distance	HR
Weather	Calories	Shoes	Other
Route		Run Type	

Friday

Time	Pace	Distance	HR
Weather	Calories	Shoes	Other
Route		Run Type	

Saturday

Time	Pace	Distance	HR
Weather	Calories	Shoes	Other
Route		Run Type	

Sunday

Time	Pace	Distance	HR
Weather	Calories	Shoes	Other
Route		Run Type	

Notes

Week Starting _____

Monday			
Time	Pace	Distance	HR
Weather	Calories	Shoes	Other
Route		Run Type	

Tuesday			
Time	Pace	Distance	HR
Weather	Calories	Shoes	Other
Route		Run Type	

Wednesday			
Time	Pace	Distance	HR
Weather	Calories	Shoes	Other
Route		Run Type	

Thursday			
Time	Pace	Distance	HR
Weather	Calories	Shoes	Other
Route		Run Type	

Friday			
Time	Pace	Distance	HR
Weather	Calories	Shoes	Other
Route		Run Type	

Saturday			
Time	Pace	Distance	HR
Weather	Calories	Shoes	Other
Route		Run Type	

Sunday			
Time	Pace	Distance	HR
Weather	Calories	Shoes	Other
Route		Run Type	

Notes

Week Starting _____

Monday			
Time	Pace	Distance	HR
Weather	Calories	Shoes	Other
Route		Run Type	

Tuesday			
Time	Pace	Distance	HR
Weather	Calories	Shoes	Other
Route		Run Type	

Wednesday			
Time	Pace	Distance	HR
Weather	Calories	Shoes	Other
Route		Run Type	

Thursday			
Time	Pace	Distance	HR
Weather	Calories	Shoes	Other
Route		Run Type	

Friday

Time	Pace	Distance	HR
Weather	Calories	Shoes	Other
Route		Run Type	

Saturday

Time	Pace	Distance	HR
Weather	Calories	Shoes	Other
Route		Run Type	

Sunday

Time	Pace	Distance	HR
Weather	Calories	Shoes	Other
Route		Run Type	

Notes

Week Starting _____

Monday

Time	Pace	Distance	HR
Weather	Calories	Shoes	Other
Route		Run Type	

Tuesday

Time	Pace	Distance	HR
Weather	Calories	Shoes	Other
Route		Run Type	

Wednesday

Time	Pace	Distance	HR
Weather	Calories	Shoes	Other
Route		Run Type	

Thursday

Time	Pace	Distance	HR
Weather	Calories	Shoes	Other
Route		Run Type	

Friday			
Time	Pace	Distance	HR
Weather	Calories	Shoes	Other
Route		Run Type	

Saturday			
Time	Pace	Distance	HR
Weather	Calories	Shoes	Other
Route		Run Type	

Sunday			
Time	Pace	Distance	HR
Weather	Calories	Shoes	Other
Route		Run Type	

Notes

Week Starting _____

Monday			
Time	Pace	Distance	HR
Weather	Calories	Shoes	Other
Route		Run Type	

Tuesday			
Time	Pace	Distance	HR
Weather	Calories	Shoes	Other
Route		Run Type	

Wednesday			
Time	Pace	Distance	HR
Weather	Calories	Shoes	Other
Route		Run Type	

Thursday			
Time	Pace	Distance	HR
Weather	Calories	Shoes	Other
Route		Run Type	

Friday

Time	Pace	Distance	HR
Weather	Calories	Shoes	Other
Route		Run Type	

Saturday

Time	Pace	Distance	HR
Weather	Calories	Shoes	Other
Route		Run Type	

Sunday

Time	Pace	Distance	HR
Weather	Calories	Shoes	Other
Route		Run Type	

Notes

Week Starting _____

Monday			
Time	Pace	Distance	HR
Weather	Calories	Shoes	Other
Route		Run Type	

Tuesday			
Time	Pace	Distance	HR
Weather	Calories	Shoes	Other
Route		Run Type	

Wednesday			
Time	Pace	Distance	HR
Weather	Calories	Shoes	Other
Route		Run Type	

Thursday			
Time	Pace	Distance	HR
Weather	Calories	Shoes	Other
Route		Run Type	

Friday

Time	Pace	Distance	HR
Weather	Calories	Shoes	Other
Route		Run Type	

Saturday

Time	Pace	Distance	HR
Weather	Calories	Shoes	Other
Route		Run Type	

Sunday

Time	Pace	Distance	HR
Weather	Calories	Shoes	Other
Route		Run Type	

Notes

Week Starting _____

Monday			
Time	Pace	Distance	HR
Weather	Calories	Shoes	Other
Route		Run Type	

Tuesday			
Time	Pace	Distance	HR
Weather	Calories	Shoes	Other
Route		Run Type	

Wednesday			
Time	Pace	Distance	HR
Weather	Calories	Shoes	Other
Route		Run Type	

Thursday			
Time	Pace	Distance	HR
Weather	Calories	Shoes	Other
Route		Run Type	

Friday

Time	Pace	Distance	HR
Weather	Calories	Shoes	Other
Route		Run Type	

Saturday

Time	Pace	Distance	HR
Weather	Calories	Shoes	Other
Route		Run Type	

Sunday

Time	Pace	Distance	HR
Weather	Calories	Shoes	Other
Route		Run Type	

Notes

Week Starting _____

Monday			
Time	Pace	Distance	HR
Weather	Calories	Shoes	Other
Route		Run Type	

Tuesday			
Time	Pace	Distance	HR
Weather	Calories	Shoes	Other
Route		Run Type	

Wednesday			
Time	Pace	Distance	HR
Weather	Calories	Shoes	Other
Route		Run Type	

Thursday			
Time	Pace	Distance	HR
Weather	Calories	Shoes	Other
Route		Run Type	

Friday

Time	Pace	Distance	HR
Weather	Calories	Shoes	Other
Route		Run Type	

Saturday

Time	Pace	Distance	HR
Weather	Calories	Shoes	Other
Route		Run Type	

Sunday

Time	Pace	Distance	HR
Weather	Calories	Shoes	Other
Route		Run Type	

Notes

Week Starting _____

Monday			
Time	Pace	Distance	HR
Weather	Calories	Shoes	Other
Route		Run Type	

Tuesday			
Time	Pace	Distance	HR
Weather	Calories	Shoes	Other
Route		Run Type	

Wednesday			
Time	Pace	Distance	HR
Weather	Calories	Shoes	Other
Route		Run Type	

Thursday			
Time	Pace	Distance	HR
Weather	Calories	Shoes	Other
Route		Run Type	

Friday			
Time	Pace	Distance	HR
Weather	Calories	Shoes	Other
Route		Run Type	

Saturday			
Time	Pace	Distance	HR
Weather	Calories	Shoes	Other
Route		Run Type	

Sunday			
Time	Pace	Distance	HR
Weather	Calories	Shoes	Other
Route		Run Type	

Notes

Week Starting _____

Monday			
Time	Pace	Distance	HR
Weather	Calories	Shoes	Other
Route		Run Type	

Tuesday			
Time	Pace	Distance	HR
Weather	Calories	Shoes	Other
Route		Run Type	

Wednesday			
Time	Pace	Distance	HR
Weather	Calories	Shoes	Other
Route		Run Type	

Thursday			
Time	Pace	Distance	HR
Weather	Calories	Shoes	Other
Route		Run Type	

Friday

Time	Pace	Distance	HR
Weather	Calories	Shoes	Other
Route		Run Type	

Saturday

Time	Pace	Distance	HR
Weather	Calories	Shoes	Other
Route		Run Type	

Sunday

Time	Pace	Distance	HR
Weather	Calories	Shoes	Other
Route		Run Type	

Notes

Week Starting _____

Monday			
Time	Pace	Distance	HR
Weather	Calories	Shoes	Other
Route		Run Type	

Tuesday			
Time	Pace	Distance	HR
Weather	Calories	Shoes	Other
Route		Run Type	

Wednesday			
Time	Pace	Distance	HR
Weather	Calories	Shoes	Other
Route		Run Type	

Thursday			
Time	Pace	Distance	HR
Weather	Calories	Shoes	Other
Route		Run Type	

Friday			
Time	Pace	Distance	HR
Weather	Calories	Shoes	Other
Route		Run Type	

Saturday			
Time	Pace	Distance	HR
Weather	Calories	Shoes	Other
Route		Run Type	

Sunday			
Time	Pace	Distance	HR
Weather	Calories	Shoes	Other
Route		Run Type	

Notes

Week Starting _____

Monday			
Time	Pace	Distance	HR
Weather	Calories	Shoes	Other
Route		Run Type	

Tuesday			
Time	Pace	Distance	HR
Weather	Calories	Shoes	Other
Route		Run Type	

Wednesday			
Time	Pace	Distance	HR
Weather	Calories	Shoes	Other
Route		Run Type	

Thursday			
Time	Pace	Distance	HR
Weather	Calories	Shoes	Other
Route		Run Type	

Friday			
Time	Pace	Distance	HR
Weather	Calories	Shoes	Other
Route		Run Type	

Saturday			
Time	Pace	Distance	HR
Weather	Calories	Shoes	Other
Route		Run Type	

Sunday			
Time	Pace	Distance	HR
Weather	Calories	Shoes	Other
Route		Run Type	

Notes

Week Starting _____

Monday			
Time	Pace	Distance	HR
Weather	Calories	Shoes	Other
Route		Run Type	

Tuesday			
Time	Pace	Distance	HR
Weather	Calories	Shoes	Other
Route		Run Type	

Wednesday			
Time	Pace	Distance	HR
Weather	Calories	Shoes	Other
Route		Run Type	

Thursday			
Time	Pace	Distance	HR
Weather	Calories	Shoes	Other
Route		Run Type	

Friday			
Time	Pace	Distance	HR
Weather	Calories	Shoes	Other
Route		Run Type	

Saturday			
Time	Pace	Distance	HR
Weather	Calories	Shoes	Other
Route		Run Type	

Sunday			
Time	Pace	Distance	HR
Weather	Calories	Shoes	Other
Route		Run Type	

Notes

Week Starting _____

Monday			
Time	Pace	Distance	HR
Weather	Calories	Shoes	Other
Route		Run Type	

Tuesday			
Time	Pace	Distance	HR
Weather	Calories	Shoes	Other
Route		Run Type	

Wednesday			
Time	Pace	Distance	HR
Weather	Calories	Shoes	Other
Route		Run Type	

Thursday			
Time	Pace	Distance	HR
Weather	Calories	Shoes	Other
Route		Run Type	

Friday

Time	Pace	Distance	HR
Weather	Calories	Shoes	Other
Route		Run Type	

Saturday

Time	Pace	Distance	HR
Weather	Calories	Shoes	Other
Route		Run Type	

Sunday

Time	Pace	Distance	HR
Weather	Calories	Shoes	Other
Route		Run Type	

Notes

Week Starting _____

Monday			
Time	Pace	Distance	HR
Weather	Calories	Shoes	Other
Route		Run Type	

Tuesday			
Time	Pace	Distance	HR
Weather	Calories	Shoes	Other
Route		Run Type	

Wednesday			
Time	Pace	Distance	HR
Weather	Calories	Shoes	Other
Route		Run Type	

Thursday			
Time	Pace	Distance	HR
Weather	Calories	Shoes	Other
Route		Run Type	

Friday			
Time	Pace	Distance	HR
Weather	Calories	Shoes	Other
Route		Run Type	

Saturday			
Time	Pace	Distance	HR
Weather	Calories	Shoes	Other
Route		Run Type	

Sunday			
Time	Pace	Distance	HR
Weather	Calories	Shoes	Other
Route		Run Type	

Notes

Week Starting _____

Monday			
Time	Pace	Distance	HR
Weather	Calories	Shoes	Other
Route		Run Type	

Tuesday			
Time	Pace	Distance	HR
Weather	Calories	Shoes	Other
Route		Run Type	

Wednesday			
Time	Pace	Distance	HR
Weather	Calories	Shoes	Other
Route		Run Type	

Thursday			
Time	Pace	Distance	HR
Weather	Calories	Shoes	Other
Route		Run Type	

Friday			
Time	Pace	Distance	HR
Weather	Calories	Shoes	Other
Route		Run Type	

Saturday			
Time	Pace	Distance	HR
Weather	Calories	Shoes	Other
Route		Run Type	

Sunday			
Time	Pace	Distance	HR
Weather	Calories	Shoes	Other
Route		Run Type	

Notes

Made in the USA
Middletown, DE
06 March 2021